Kitchen Cabinet Medicine –

Anti-inflammatory Edition

Using the ingredients in your kitchen to reverse
chronic inflammation

By Deb Maselli

Medical Disclaimer:

The content of this book is provided for general informational purposes only and is not intended as, or a substitute for, professional medical advice. Do not use the information in this book for diagnosing or treating any medical or health condition. If you have or suspect you have a medical problem, promptly contact your professional healthcare provider. Always ask your health care provider before taking any new supplement.

Table of Contents

Introduction

These days, there is a pill or a capsule for whatever ails you. But the most powerful medicine has always been right in your kitchen cabinet. The most powerful medicine is low cost, easy to incorporate into a busy life, does not require a total re-haul of diet and lifestyle and does not need a prescription.

Chronic inflammation is running rampant throughout the developed world. Never before have we seen this virtual mushroom cloud of infirmities. If you or someone you know has suffered from arthritis, asthma, gum disease, heart disease, diabetes, stomach ulcer, depression, leaky gut, hay fever, irritable bowel syndrome, acne, psoriasis, Grave's disease, fibromyalgia, Addison's, Alzheimer's, Lupus, gall bladder attacks, cancer, and the list goes on and on — you have seen the effects of chronic inflammation.

We have become a nation of people who have 'conditions.' We no longer find it strange that so many commercials on television feature smiling people with chronic ailments. People in the prime of their life, doomed to carry around catheters or glucose testers or inhalers everywhere they go. We no longer blink at the television announcer mentioning that one of the side effects of the medication being hawked to cure us may be death. The announcer suggests that you talk to your doctor about this medication and find out if it is right for you. After all, not everybody who takes this medication dies.

These medications, which have become a booming business for pharmaceutical companies, are treating conditions and diseases caused by chronic, low-grade inflammation.

But is chronic inflammation and the diseases it brings on the body just an unfortunate side effect of modern living? To a great degree, yes it is. Chronic inflammation is most definitely a side effect of our modern world. Does that mean if we want to live a long, healthy, pain-free life we should move to a mountain top and become a hermit, only subsisting on organic foods?

Well, that would be one approach. Another approach is far simpler. Inflammatory substances are cumulative. It is not necessary to avoid all substances with inflammatory properties. In fact, it would be impossible. Even some nutrient-dense, healthful foods are slightly inflammatory. But if you are able to tip the balance even slightly in favor of anti-inflammatory, you have won the inflammation war and prevented chronic conditions and diseases down the road. Adding super anti-inflammatories in small amounts on a daily basis helps to counterbalance the damaging inflammatory properties of everything else you consumed or were exposed to during the day.

The result? Chronic ailments begin to heal. That includes our number one chronic ailment - obesity. Fat cells, particularly around the waist, set off a chain of events that promote inflammation, promote fat storage and promote the increase of fat cells. You were wondering why it was easy to lose weight at twenty, but now it seems impossible? A slowing metabolism is only part of the equation. Inflammation is encouraging your body to hold on to fat, rather than release it.

What is so insidious about inflammation is that it is silent and invisible. It does its damaging work for years before a person becomes aware of the damage through a symptom like arthritis or heart disease or cancer. If there is anything that baby boomers can contribute to future generations, it is the example of what happens to a body that has consumed too much inflammatory food, without balancing it with anti-inflammatory food. The baby boomers were the generation that grew up on packaged, processed food, before anybody knew that trans-fats will kill you and sugar provokes inflammation. The boomers are the generation of lab rats that are now paying the price for innovations in convenience, and they are lining the pockets of the pharmaceutical companies while they suffer.

The state of food in our country is both disheartening and heartening. It is disheartening that we are still faced with major food manufacturers and fast food chains launching quite disingenuous campaigns to convince Americans that their products are providing real health benefits. That what was once a cookie is now a "breakfast bar" and that's okay. That what was once a piece of fruit is now a jell-like substance in a cardboard container, and that's okay. That the drive-through can provide real nutrition.

That a commercially prepared smoothie full of sugar is good for you.

On the other hand, we have never had so much choice at such low cost and there is an emerging industry of food manufacturers who are honestly seeking to provide healthful, tastes-good, choices within the confines of mass production. As well, it is heartening that the American consumer grows savvier by the minute and this, in turn, will push the major manufacturers to think twice before selling a product full of sugar and fat as "a great way to start the day."

I do not believe there is anything inherently wrong with junk food. I do not believe it should be regulated or controlled, other than providing clear nutrition labeling. After all, we are a nation of freedom of choice, and frankly, there is nothing more tedious than a health nut, holy roller who is not satisfied with making their own food choices, but want to make yours as well. But if we know that what we are consuming is junk, and we know that it causes inflammation in the body, which in turn leads to chronic diseases and conditions, then we can consume with our eyes wide open and take steps to rebalance the inflammatory load without unduly disrupting our lifestyle.

If you are now in your twenties, you probably eat what you want, drink as much soda as you like and feel pretty good. The idea that the damage is being done and you will pay for it later probably doesn't cause much of a blip on the radar. But look at the adults around you in their fifties, sixties and seventies. How are they doing? Anybody using a cane? Anybody testing their glucose every day? How about adding a few highly anti-inflammatory foods to your diet without giving up all the things you love and end up looking and feeling like thirty when you turn fifty? That's a better future.

Or perhaps you are older, you are one of those baby boomers, and are feeling the effects of decades of inflammatory foods and toxins. Is it too late? No. Is it most definitely not too late. By reversing inflammation now, you can reverse much of the damage that has been done and you will feel better than you have in a very long time.

Or perhaps you are a parent, desperately trying to ensure your child's healthy future, but stymied by all the temptations a young person faces throughout the day. You can't follow them everywhere. You can't control everything they eat. And do you really have the heart to say no to cake at a birthday party or tell them Halloween has been cancelled? Do you have the energy and time to declare your family will NEVER eat fast food?

Thanks to modern research on inflammation – what causes it and how we can counteract it – it is possible to live in the modern world, and enjoy modern world conveniences, without suffering the devastating effects of chronic inflammation.

This book will explain how to do just that. You don't have to become a vegetarian or drink green smoothies or give up red meat and dessert if that's not for you. By tweaking some of your favorite meals, you can undo the damage of chronic inflammation.

Because the most powerful medicine has always been right in your kitchen cabinet.

Chapter One

What is chronic inflammation?

Inflammation, in and of itself, is not inherently bad. It is the body's very effective response to a perceived threat. Chronic inflammation occurs when the body's effective response to a perceived threat has run amok and is now itself causing damage.

The easiest way to picture inflammation in the body is to imagine a stove top burner. Acute inflammation would cause the flame to rise and burn brightly. But only for a short amount of time. A stubbed toe sends the fire shooting up. A few days later, the fire is out. But in chronic inflammation, the stove has been left on low. Permanently.

Once the stove has been left on low, an environment has been created in the body where the immune system will remain on high alert at all times.

A healthy immune system is a finely tuned warrior. It lays in wait for incoming invaders. When it senses an attack, it launches an effective counter-attack. When the invader is defeated, the healthy immune system takes a well-earned rest.

But a compromised immune system no longer knows what an invader looks like. A compromised immune system fires off chemical weapons at any and all comers, all day long.

Chronic, low grade inflammation can occur for years before a person notices they have a problem. Unfortunately, the first sign of chronic inflammation is often a debilitating condition that severely compromises the subject's quality of life, or a disease that may actually end the subject's life.

Chapter Two

What causes inflammation?

Chronic inflammation is so rampant today because the causes of inflammation are so prevalent. Here's the list:

Alcohol – Alcohol can contribute to a leaky gut. Once toxins are released into the blood stream, the immune system generates an inflammatory response to attempt to mitigate the damage.

Animal fats – Animal fats disrupt the balance of friendly gut bacteria and promote inflammation.

Food sensitivities – A food that might otherwise carry health benefits, like organic milk, can cause inflammation in people who have a sensitivity to it. A person who has a strong reaction to a particular food group is actually in a better spot than those that only have a mild reaction. The strong reactors simply eliminate the food causing them a problem. The mild reactors may not be able to identify that they even have a food sensitivity or be able to identify what particular food is causing the problem. Anyone experiencing chronic pain or fatigue or bowel issues would be well-served to keep a food diary for a few weeks and periodically remove and add back different food groups to identify the culprit.

Genetics – Unfortunately, even if you do everything right (if that were possible, which it is not) you can still suffer from chronic inflammation. A gene has been identified that acts to clear away cells that have been unduly stressed. Mutations of that gene lead to less effective clearing, which leads to inflammation.

Gluten – those with Celiac disease have a particular sensitivity to gluten and this sensitivity provokes a very definite immune response, leading to inflammation. It is speculated that many people who do not have Celiac may have a less intense sensitivity which provokes chronic low grade inflammation.

Gum disease – gum disease is a low grade infection. As such, the immune system kicks into gear and stays there until the bad bacteria is physically removed from the teeth and the gum reattaches more firmly to the teeth.

Imbalanced gut bacteria – When helpful gut bacteria are overwhelmed by bad bacteria, the lining of the digestive tract may become compromised. This introduces foreign toxins into the rest of the body and the immune system causes inflammation in an attempt to rectify the situation.

Lack of moderate exercise – A sedentary lifestyle promotes inflammation, moderate exercise fights inflammation. It is helpful to note that strenuous exercise also promotes inflammation in the short term. Those individuals wishing to begin exercising to reduce inflammation are advised to begin slowly.

Lack of sleep – Similar to the stress response, less than six hours of sleep per night deregulates the body's immune system, causing inflammation. Young, healthy adults with no other risk factors raised their risk of stroke by almost five percent, just from a lack of sleep.

Metabolic Syndrome - Chronic inflammation from other factors such as obesity or stress cause metabolic syndrome to develop. High blood pressure, high triglycerides, high cholesterol, and high blood sugar then contribute to further inflammation.

MSG – the link between MSG and inflammation is documented, though the mechanism is still unknown.

Obesity – The link between obesity and inflammation is clear. The exact mechanism is still up for debate. One theory proposes that fat tissue signals the body's immune system that something is wrong. The immune system kicks into high gear, causing inflammation. When the fat tissue remains, so does the inflammation.

Omega 6 overload – Omega 6 and Omega 3 should be balanced. However, in the standard American diet, Omega 6 is far too abundant and Omega 3 much too scant. This promotes an inflammatory state in the body.

Smoking – the toxins in cigarette smoke are proven inflammatory triggers.

Stress – Prolonged stress interferes with the hormone cortisol. Cortisol regulates the immune system. Once this regulation has been compromised, the immune system is no longer regulated and inflammation results. This is why one person only gets the sniffles, while another person exposed to same cold virus gets a full blown head cold. The inflammatory response is not being regulated properly by cortisol.

Sugar – Sugar sends signals to the immune system to kick into high gear.

Toxins – phthalates found in beauty and personal care products, Bisphenol A found in plastics, mercury, cigarette smoke, household chemicals, air pollution, lawn and garden chemicals, bacteria, mold – we are surrounded by toxins. Once the toxin tipping point has been reached in the body, the immune system remains constantly active, resulting in chronic inflammation.

Trans fats - Trans fats damage the linings of cells and the immune system kicks in to attempt to repair, creating ongoing inflammation.

Vitamin A deficiency – Though it is rare in the developed world, a deficiency in Vitamin A causes a whole host of symptoms and creates an inflammatory state in the body.

White bread – Refined flour is quickly broken down into sugar and provokes the same inflammatory response.

Chapter Three

How do I know if I have chronic inflammation?

You won't necessarily know that you have chronic inflammation. Especially if you are young, symptoms may not have presented themselves yet. However, chronic pain, chronic fatigue, chronic bowel issues, chronic allergies and chronic asthma are all markers for chronic inflammation. In general, it is probably safe to assume that if you are living in the modern world and are not compensating for the inflammatory triggers you expose your body to on a daily basis, you already have chronic, low grade inflammation.

There is a test available that can measure inflammation. The blood test that measures C-Reactive Protein is a reliable indicator of inflammation. The test is usually reserved for patients suspected of heart disease, but it is a simple blood test and there is no reason your doctor couldn't order it for you. If you ask.

Another reliable away to assess inflammation is to add super anti-inflammatories into your diet and then monitor how you feel. Most people feel a surge in energy and notice that aches and pains they have become accustomed to have receded or disappeared. Weight becomes easier to lose. Skin eruptions clear up. A sense of well-being returns to the body.

Chapter Four

How do Anti-inflammatory foods work?

Each day, the human body is exposed to both inflammatory substances and anti-inflammatory substances. The amount of inflammation the body is subjected to, whether through food, lack of exercise, obesity, smoking and all the other reasons previously noted, is the body's inflammation load. This inflammation load can be cancelled out by an equal or greater anti-inflammation load.

Imagine the scales of justice. On the inflammation side is the cheeseburger you had for lunch, the stress you experienced in an afternoon meeting, a missed day at the gym because you overslept and lack of sleep because you were out late the night before, which is why you overslept in the first place. All of that needs to be balanced on the anti-inflammation side of the scale.

Since we are talking about imaginary scales, there is no hard and fast formula for calculating what or how much to take in on the anti-inflammation side of the scales. Even if you were to use numerical assignments to denote the degree of inflammatory or anti-inflammatory effects, measuring inflammation load is an imperfect science at best.

It is helpful, however, to understand to what degree particular substances are inflammatory or anti-inflammatory. The best known system for quantifying anti-inflammatory qualities is the IF (Inflammatory Factor Rating TM) ratings given by Monica Reinagel, http://inflammationfactor.com/

But, as there is simply no way to account for inflammatory factors you may not even be aware of, it is best to try to overbalance the scales toward anti-inflammatory. Take the above example – what if, on top of the other factors promoting inflammation, a mercury filling is leaching, unbeknownst to the person trying to figure out their inflammation load?

By making simple switches and additions to your normal diet, you can increase the likelihood that your anti-inflammatory load is tipping the scales in your favor.

Chapter Five

Anti-inflammatory foods

The following list of foods and ingredients can be added to a normal diet to counterbalance exposure to, and ingestion of, inflammatory substances. This guide is not meant to suggest that a person need transform his or herself into an organic vegetarian who meditates instead of eats snacks. Bravo to those people who live a strictly healthy lifestyle.

But then, there are the rest of us.

The rest of us make mistakes, have slip ups and indulge in distinctly non-healthy food and life-style choices because we like it and don't really want to give up the small joys in life. The rest of us can battle chronic inflammation by making changes that do not create a hardship or a sense of deprivation. We are not looking for perfection; we are just looking to tip the scales in our favor.

One of the interesting things to note about anti-inflammatory foods is that results are cumulative. So for instance, doubling the amount of a moderately anti-inflammatory substance will likely push that substance's effect on the body into the strongly anti-inflammatory range.

Each item is listed by amount and by the anti-inflammatory punch it provides. Substances are graded as highly anti-inflammatory, moderately anti-inflammatory, slightly anti-inflammatory and neutral. The anti-inflammatory items will counteract the inflammation the body has been subjected to on a daily basis. As for the neutral items, these provide other health benefits that assist in controlling inflammation and do not contribute to inflammation so end up coming out on the positive side. Also, it is almost always the case that when you add a neutral food, you have removed an inflammatory food, tipping the scales in the right direction.

Acerola cherries,1 C   Strongly anti-inflammatory

Almond butter, 1C   Strongly anti-inflammatory

Almonds, 1C   Strongly anti-inflammatory

Anchovies, 1oz   Strongly anti-inflammatory

Atlantic herring 1 fillet Strongly anti-inflammatory

Avocado oil, 1oz   Moderately anti-inflammatory

Avocado, 1   Moderately anti-inflammatory

Basil, dried, 1T	Mildly anti-inflammatory
Black pepper, 1 dash	Neutral
Blueberries, 1oz	Neutral
Brazil nuts, 1oz	Moderately anti-inflammatory
Broccoli, 1 C	Mildly anti-inflammatory
Cardamom, 1t	Neutral
Carrots, 1C	Moderately anti-inflammatory
Cashew butter, 1T	Mildly anti-inflammatory
Cauliflower, 1C	Mildly anti-inflammatory
Caviar, 1T	Strongly anti-inflammatory
Cayenne, 1T	Strongly anti-inflammatory
Chamomile, 1 C tea	Mildly anti-inflammatory
Chia seeds, 1oz	Mildly anti-inflammatory

Chili powder, 1T	Strongly anti-inflammatory
Cilantro , 1 T	Mildly anti-inflammatory
Cinnamon, 1T	Neutral
Cloves, 1T	Neutral
Cocoa powder, 1T	Neutral
Collards, 1 C	Strongly anti-inflammatory
Cranberries, 1C	Mildly anti-inflammatory
Currants, 1 C	Mildly anti-inflammatory
Curry powder, 1T	Strongly anti-inflammatory
Extra virgin olive oil,1C	Strongly anti-inflammatory
Garlic powder ,1T	Strongly anti-inflammatory
Garlic, 1T	Strongly anti-inflammatory
Ginger, 1T	Strongly anti-inflammatory

Green tea, 1 C	Strongly anti-inflammatory
Guava , 1 C	Moderately anti-inflammatory
Halibut, 1 Fillet	Strongly anti-inflammatory
Hazelnuts, 1oz	Moderately anti-inflammatory
Hot sauce, 1t	Strongly anti-inflammatory
Jalapeno pepper, 1oz	Moderately anti-inflammatory
Kale, 1 C	Strongly anti-inflammatory
Kelp, 1T	Mildly anti-inflammatory
Lemon zest, 1T	Mildly anti-inflammatory
Macadamia, 1 C	Strongly anti-inflammatory
Mackerel, 1 Fillet	Strongly anti-inflammatory
Marjoram, 1T	Mildly anti-inflammatory
Melon, cantaloupe 1 C	Mildly anti-inflammatory

Mozzarella, 1 C	Mildly anti-inflammatory
Mustard seed, 1T	Mildly anti-inflammatory
Nutmeg, 1T	Mildly anti-inflammatory
Olives, 1	Mildly anti-inflammatory
Onion powder, 1T	Strongly anti-inflammatory
Onions, 1 C	Strongly anti-inflammatory
Oregano, 1T	Mildly anti-inflammatory
Oysters, 3oz	Strongly anti-inflammatory
Papaya, 1 C	Mildly anti-inflammatory
Parsley, 1T	Mildly anti-inflammatory
Peanut butter, 2T	Mildly anti-inflammatory
Pecans, 1 C	Moderately anti-inflammatory
Pineapple, 1 C	Mildly anti-inflammatory

Pumpkin, 1 C   Strongly anti-inflammatory

Rainbow trout 1 Fillet Strongly anti-inflammatory

Raspberry, 1 C   Mildly anti-inflammatory

Red pepper flakes, 1T Strongly anti-inflammatory

Rosemary, 1 T   Neutral

Sage, 1T   Mildly anti-inflammatory

Salsa, 1 C   Mildly anti-inflammatory

Spinach, 1 C   Mildly anti-inflammatory

Strawberries, 1 C   Mildly anti-inflammatory

Sweet potato, 1 C   Strongly anti-inflammatory

Thyme, 1T   Mildly anti-inflammatory

Turmeric, 1T   Strongly anti-inflammatory

Wild caught salmon1filletStrongly anti-inflammatory

Chapter Six

Simple switches with big payoff

These small changes to day to day eating really add up. Removing an inflammatory and replacing it with an anti-inflammatory has a positive, double-whammy effect. For example, 1T of regular corn oil has an inflammatory factor of forty-nine. 1T of avocado oil has an anti-inflammatory factor of 68. Were you to continue using 1T of regular corn oil, and simply added 1T of avocado oil, you would cancel out the corn oil and still be ahead by a factor of nineteen on the anti-inflammatory side of the scales. But, if you switch the 1T of corn oil for 1T of avocado oil you have both removed an inflammatory substance from the inflammation side of the scales and added an anti-inflammatory substance to the anti-inflammation side of the scales, leaving you a factor of one hundred and seventeen on the positive side of the scales. That surplus can then be used to counteract something else you ingested or were exposed to that is inflammatory.

Remove sugar and replace with Stevia

Remove common cooking oils and switch to avocado oil

Remove salad dressing made with vegetable oil and switch to olive oil

Remove regular milk and switch to organic milk

Remove yogurt and switch to kefir

Remove non-organic beef and switch to free range

Remove processed meat and switch to non-processed meat

Remove refined grains and switch to whole grains

Remove aspartame and other fake sweeteners and switch to Stevia

Remove MSG and switch to flavorful herbs and spices

Remove white potato and switch to sweet potato

Remove white wine and other alcohol and switch to red wine

Remove milk chocolate and switch to 70 percent dark chocolate

Remove American cheese and switch to mozzarella

Chapter Seven

The Anti-inflammatory Superstars

Adding just one of the following ingredients to your daily diet will have a profound effect on inflammation. These ingredients can be up to ten times higher than the baseline for a strongly anti-inflammatory food. As such, simply adding one of these ingredients to your diet on a daily basis can cancel out a whole host of inflammatory sins.

Anchovies

Caviar

Cayenne pepper

Garlic

Ginger

Olive oil

Onions

Salmon

Turmeric

Chapter Eight

Anti-inflammatory vitamins and supplements

Before adding any new supplement, consult with your doctor. Some supplements are not compatible with certain medications and conditions.

Catechins – Catechins are a substance found in green tea. Catechins are documented to prevent diseases that result from chronic inflammation, like cancer, heart disease and Alzheimer's.

Citrus Bio-flavanoids – Bio-flavanoids are found in citrus fruits. In supplement form, bio-flavanoids are often combined with Vitamin C to promote absorption. Bio-flavanoids inhibit inflammation and are particularly helpful for people suffering from inflammation involving joints, like arthritis.

Fish oil omega 3 – Fish oil supplements contain an essential fatty acid called EPA, which assists in calming inflammation. The mechanism through which it does so is ingenious. The components of fish oil essentially work inside the body's cells, prompting the cells to produce more calming chemicals into the body. This is particularly helpful in obese subjects, as the extra pounds are constantly shooting off signals to encourage inflammation. The suggested dose for fish oil varies widely and you should consult your doctor about what dose would be appropriate. When purchasing fish oil, it is vital to buy a high-quality product free from mercury or other contaminants.

Ginger – Ginger is a potent anti-inflammatory and can be taken in capsule form. Though it is best known for soothing upset stomach and treating motion sickness, ginger can be enormously helpful in controlling body-wide inflammation and can resolve many digestive issues. It is particularly helpful in treating chronic bloating after eating.

Kelp – Kelp contains the substance fucoidan. Fucoidan has been proven to control inflammation and may prevent certain cancers. As with fish oil, buy a high quality supplement that is guaranteed to be toxin free. It won't do your body much good if the kelp has been harvested from contaminated waters. Avoid supplementing with kelp snacks, as they are generally overloaded with salt.

Magnesium – Magnesium is a vital mineral and long known to control inflammation. A majority of Americans do not consume the recommended levels of magnesium. If supplementing with magnesium, buy a high quality brand that is a blend of different types of magnesium. Never buy a version that is only magnesium oxide; that type of magnesium is usually the cheapest, but your body will not absorb it well and it will likely cause diarrhea.

Probiotic b infantis – Ingestion of the probiotic b infantis has been shown to have a positive effect on tests for C-Reactive protein. As discussed earlier, C-Reactive protein is a routine test done by doctors to assess an individual's inflammatory state.

Quercetin – Quercetin is a type of bio-flavanoid found in such diverse foods as apples, tea, onions and red wine. Quercetin is recognized as being extremely effective at controlling inflammation, easing the pain of arthritis and reducing the size of some cancer tumors.

Turmeric – It is suggested earlier in this book to add turmeric to your diet. This mega-anti-inflammatory is available in supplement form and is a cornerstone of Ayurvedic medicine. Turmeric is so effective at fighting inflammation that, unless you fall in love with the spice and plan on cooking with it often, it would be well worth considering adding it as a supplement.

Vitamin C – Many people with chronic inflammation are deficient in Vitamin C. Adding Vitamin C may assist the body in calming inflammation.

Zinc – Mild zinc deficiency often goes hand in hand with chronic inflammation. Whether the zinc deficiency is actually causing or contributing to the inflammation is not clear, but what is documented is that supplementation of small amounts of zinc have a very interesting effect. Most anti-inflammatories suppress the immune system's over-response to perceived threats. Zinc appears to repair the immune system response. So, rather than suppression, there is correction.

And one more thing to do – FLOSS!

Physically removing bacteria from the teeth prevents gum disease. Gum disease is highly inflammatory and has been implicated as a culprit in heart disease. If you do not floss because your gums are sore or you find you cannot easily pull the floss between your teeth, see a dentist and have a thorough cleaning. A cleaning should resolve those issues. If you, like many Americans, have not seen a dentist recently because you are terrified of the dentist, take heart. Dentistry has improved leaps and bounds from just ten years ago, particularly in the area of patient comfort. Many dentists are able to knock you out for even just a cleaning. If in doubt, take the first step. Call for a consultation in which you will simply arrive at the office and speak to the dentist. Do not be afraid of insisting that the dentist may only use a mirror to examine your teeth, no touching allowed. It is not necessary for a dentist to poke and prod to see how much a tooth or your gums hurt. An X-ray will suffice to look at damage, and once you are sedated, the dentist can poke and prod all they like. Feeling comfortable and trusting your dentist is vital to patients who are afraid of dentistry. Those patients will be better served seeing a dentist who specializes in pain-free dentistry. Once you have restored your teeth and gums to health, use floss. Water irrigation systems are fine to use in conjunction with floss if you particularly like them, but they in no way take the place of the physical action of floss against tooth.

And finally, life is meant to be lived. There is no reason to hide atop a mountain, subsisting on organic food. Your body would love you for it, but it would be an unsatisfying life. Get out there, have fun, eat some junk when you feel like it. Just remember to counterbalance the junk with the anti-inflammatories right in your kitchen cabinet.

More From Deb Maselli

Coming Soon: Kitchen Cabinet Medicine – Antioxidant Edition

Available Now:

Beat the Bloat – Saying Goodbye to Stomach Bloating Forever

http://www.amazon.com/Beat-Bloat-Bloating-Forever-ebook/dp/B00E7XWT9G

This book was written for people whose stomach bloats nearly every day, usually after eating. It is a step by step guide that explains why your stomach bloats, why you have excess gas, and how to eliminate bloating and gas by healing your digestive tract through the use of inexpensive and widely available supplements.

How does your stomach feel? Okay in the morning, but by the afternoon you look a little pregnant? You bloat after eating? Your bowel habits have become unpredictable? You used to have an iron stomach, and now you don't?

You can thank the Standard American Diet (the S.A.D) for your woes. The S.A.D. derails healthy digestion. Once the digestive tract is compromised, bloating and gas result. Even worse, the S.A.D. doesn't just compromise your digestion while you're eating it. It compromises your digestion permanently, until you take steps to undo the damage. If you're already suffering from a chronically bloated stomach, cleaning up your diet won't fix the problem. Your digestive system needs to be repaired.

Discover the simple, three step solution to healing your digestion and eliminating bloating and gas by regulating transit time, increasing efficient nutrient absorption and effectively establishing helpful bacteria. Find out why you bloat every time you eat, why slow digestive transit time contributes to the problem, how inflammation can irritate the vagus nerve, which mineral can correct transit time, how digestive enzymes work, the difference between pro and prebiotics, what fiber is really doing in there, and how vitamins and herbs can work together to repair the damage inflicted on your digestive system by the S.A.D.

This book contains the seven-day get back on track program called T.A.B. The T.A.B. formula is easy to follow, it is comprised of widely available, inexpensive supplements and does not involve a restrictive diet.

With the right supplements in the right combination, it's possible to correct the imbalances caused by the S.A.D. and eliminate bloating and gas once and for all.

I KNOW you can bring your digestive system back to a healthy state. You can do it without confining yourself to a narrow list of foods or following complicated rituals. Once you understand the three keys to healthy digestion, and how supplements work to support the three keys, you'll never suffer from bloating and gas again.

Here's to living life NOT thinking about your stomach.

www.ingramcontent.com/pod-product-compliance
Lightning Source LLC
Chambersburg PA
CBHW070840290526
45795CB00002B/935